I0830402

BE A

SUPER STAR

IN BED

Tips to Last Longer With Your Partner

I DEDICATED

THIS BOOK

TO ALL MEN

CONTENTS

<u>ACKNOWLEGEMENT</u>

All praise and adoration is due to nobody except almighty

God the lord of mankind. I praise him and glorified him

for is protections and blessings over me so far. And also

for giving me opportunities to create this small work, for

the benefit of my readers. I am also indebted to my late

father for his tremendous efforts to make my education

successful. May his gentle soul continue to rest in perfect

peace till eternity (amen). And also to my great mother

for her intensive supports on very steps I take. May she

live long to eat the fruit of her labor. This work would not

have seen the light of the day if not for the prayers,

patronage and encouragement of my readers. I thank

you all, may almighty god in his infinity mercy continue

and protect every one of us (amen).

16 Hints to Endure Longer With Your Accomplice

1. Dial back. The absolute most significant suggestion I
will at any point give you.

2. Utilize a thick condom. This can diminish your
awareness. It may not feel quite a bit better yet it will
assist you with becoming acclimated to the uplifted
excitement of genuine love making.

3**. Use Theater of the Brain and Art strategy to keep
your outlook and self-talk positive**.

4. *Make ideal circumstances*. Realize your

Circumstances for Good Sex and ensure they are

occurring.

5. *Convey.* Especially with another accomplice,

correspondence is fundamental. You are finding out

about one another's body and sentiments. Let her know

if you are on the edge.

6. Know about when you become over energized or

unfortunate and utilize Quiet Body, Quiet Brain to take

back to unwinding.

7. Appreciate long foreplay. Try not to hurry into

penetrative sex, enjoy a rich buffet of appetizers.

 8. Disregard Pornstar. Try not to attempt to perform,

flaunt or dazzle her. Simply be you.

9. Enter progressively. Try not to simply push in. Go in

leisurely and delicately, becoming accustomed to the

sensations. Make sure to utilize profound loosened up

breathing to quiet you down.

10. Stand by inside her. At the point when you are inside

her, be still for some time before you begin pushing. It

tends to be an otherworldly second. Eye to eye

connection is perfect.

11. Begin with little sluggish developments. Once more,

dial back.

12. Utilize both crushing and pushing developments.

Pushing is in and out developments. Crushing is

roundabout developments which don't slide in and out.

Crushing developments feel significantly better to both

of you yet are less invigorating to you, so you can endure

longer. I investigate this in more profundity in my

subsequent book, 1000 Adoring Pushes, to be distributed

soon.

13. Utilize the Traffic Signal framework. Attempt to

remain in GREEN however much you can and cycle all

over from Golden.

14. Utilize the huge crush and different methods from

the performance rehearses.

15. At the point when you are prepared, go with a

positive decision to discharge. At the point when you

really do discharge let it all out.

16. Pull out leisurely and delicately, remain in actual

association. Orgasmic Capturing and How to Stay away

from It with an Accomplice Orgasmic seizing happens

when a man ends up being over invigorated or over

associated with his darling's excitement and climax. As a

man you will no doubt find your accomplice's excitement

profoundly invigorating. The manner in which she moves

and inhales, the sounds she makes, the blushing of her

skin, her erect areolas, her wetness, her capacity to give

up and let endlessly go into the progression of her sexual

joy are exceptionally powerful turn-ons. This is a

delightful and an extremely rich piece of the experience

of lovemaking and sexual closeness. You are favored to

observe something genuinely otherworldly and holy. The

risk for men is that we become so centered around our

darling that we move away from our own body, our own

sentiments and our own pleasure. For certain men it is

more that he turns out to be so centered around

pleasuring his sweetheart on "giving" her a climax that he

gets a sense of ownership with his own pleasure and

fulfillment. This is specific the situation with men who

have been raised in areas of strength for an ethic. In the

tantric sexual moment too there is a propensity for men

to accept that their essential job is to love and delight the

Goddess, for example the lady. Presently this is valid, yet

just half obvious. In a decent relationship the two

accomplices get a sense of ownership with their own

pleasure while pleasuring one another. I went through a

stage where orgasmic commandeering was an issue for

me. I'm a characteristic empath. I feel others'

contemplations and feelings effectively and

straightforwardly at times to where they could cloud my

feeling of my own personality. With my sweetheart,

when she entered a truly profound degree of orgasmic

excitement, I could get so up to speed in her vivacious

delivery that I went there as well. I felt all that she felt. I

nearly turned into her. Some of the time I wound up

discharging when she is still in full stream. As a result I

came for her, yet rashly, I'd captured her climax. To take

a gander at it the alternate way round, when a lady is in

her full power, her sexual charge can be overpowering

and in a real sense hauls a discharge out of the man. So

by the day's end, it's difficult to say who has captured

whom. In a genuinely open and personal connection,

orgasmic commandeering can appear every once in a

while and can be straightforwardly investigated as a

component of the excursion towards more profound

closeness. It was this way for myself as well as my

sweetheart. The learning for me was tied in with

remaining present to my own body and my own power.

In the event that a man can remain cool and hold

presence through his darling's excitement, the two

accomplices can at last experience a significantly more

profound consolidating and give up. Working with clients

over numerous years, I have understood that orgasmic

capturing is a typical issue for men. It very well may be a

major snare while creating Ejaculatory Opportunity,

since, supposing that you are excessively centered

around your sweetheart you can lose mindfulness and

handily become over energized. The spearheading sex

advisor, the late Bernie Zeibergeld expounded on the

peculiarity of orgasmic commandeering back quite a few

years prior, despite the fact that he didn't utilize that

term. He proposed a Performance center of the Psyche

type practice where you distinctively envision your

accomplice going every one of the phases of her

excitement to an extraordinary orgasmic discharge while

rehashing the mantra: "Her energy isn't my fervor. Her

enthusiasm isn't my obsession. She's doing her thing

however I need to do my own, zeroing in on my own

sentiments" Learning Ejaculatory Opportunity with a

Substitute For men beating serious untimely discharge

issues especially where there a profound intense subject

matters included, a sexual proxy accomplice might assist

with spanning the difficult hole once again into a

wonderful personal connection. Surrogacy is a potential

way forward where a man feels a great deal of dread and

tension around closeness and connections. A substitute

accomplice is an expert specialist who fills in as a

substitute cooperate with whom to investigate and

rehearse physical and close to home closeness abilities.

The treatment might incorporate sex where this is

suitable albeit contacting, relational abilities, relationship

abilities and unwinding methods are comparably

significant. Proxies normally work related to a sex

specialist or clinician in spite of the fact that they, when

all is said and done, are generally qualified in directing

and sex. Surrogacy has been around since the 1970s as a

genuine calling in spite of the fact that there are as a

matter of fact, not very many proxies accessible to work

with clients, and hardly any sex specialists who work with

substitutes. Substitutes are not whores yet are

thoroughly prepared and caring people are in contact

with their own sexuality and proposition this work as a

mending administration. On the off chance that you feel

this sort of treatment would help you, you would

accomplish best to work with a guide or sexuality

specialist to investigate the more extensive setting of

your issues and choose if and when surrogacy would be

the correct way forward. The expense of surrogacy is

generally exceptionally high. I work with a little

organization of substitutes to whom I can allude clients

where suitable after they have work 1:1 with me on the

fundamental issues. Might I at any point go to a whore?

To start with, I need to say that I am making no ethical

judgment about the world's most established calling.

Many whores are faithful and proposition an expert

support of their clients. In this day and age prostitution

appear to fill a vital need for both their clients and

presumably for the sex laborers themselves. We would

do well to decriminalize and appropriately direct the

calling. Be that as it may, for a man wishing to conquer

untimely discharge, a visit to a whore is probably not

going to be useful. First and foremost, what whores are

selling is a dream experience not a real encounter of

lovemaking and closeness. They are selling the "sizzle"

not the "frankfurter". Besides, the dream served by

prostitution will support the propensities for Mountain

man and Mr Alpha. These are the characteristics you

really want to control, assuming that you will acquire

Ejaculatory Opportunity. Thirdly, a whore isn't prepared

in the remedial techniques that will assist you with

beating untimely discharge. At last, many whores need to

keep their experience with a client as short as could be

expected. They are capable at making you discharge

rapidly. Key bring back Home from This Part There is a

great deal in this section. You've learned: • How to

approach and converse with your accomplice about

creating ejaculatory opportunity. • How to rehearse with

a helpful accomplice to expand your Ejaculatory

Opportunity. • How to move toward things in the event that you don't have an accomplice. • The dangers of orgasmic commandeering and how to keep away from them. • When a sexual proxy accomplice is suitable.